The Vibrant Slow Cooker Delicacies

Affordable Delicious and Super Tasty

Fish for everyday meals

Donna Conway

© copyright 2021 – all rights reserved.

the content contained within this book may not be reproduced, duplicated or transmitted without direct written permission from the author or the publisher.

under no circumstances will any blame or legal responsibility be held against the publisher, or author, for any damages, reparation, or monetary loss due to the information contained within this book. either directly or indirectly.

legal notice:

this book is copyright protected. this book is only for personal use. you cannot amend, distribute, sell, use, quote or paraphrase any part, or the content within this book, without the consent of the author or publisher.

disclaimer notice:

please note the information contained within this document is for educational and entertainment purposes only. all effort has been executed to present accurate, up to date, and reliable, complete information. no warranties of any kind are declared or implied. readers acknowledge that the author is not engaging in the rendering of legal, financial, medical or professional advice. the content within this book has been derived from various sources. please consult a licensed professional before attempting any techniques outlined in this book.

by reading this document, the reader agrees that under no circumstances is the author responsible for any losses, direct or indirect, which are incurred as a result of the use of information contained within this document, including, but not limited to, — errors, omissions, or inaccuracies.

Table of Contents

- Beef Stroganoff 6
- Cabbage & Corned Beef 8
- Chipotle Barbacoa – Mexican Barbecue 10
- Corned Beef Cabbage Rolls 12
- Cube Steak 15
- Italian Meatballs & Zoodles 17
- London Broil 20
- Machaca - Mexican Pot Roast 22
- Cranberry Pork Roast 25
- Pulled Pork 27
- Balsamic Pork Tenderloin 29
- Honey Mustard Barbecue Pork Ribs 31
- Pork Chops with Broccoli 33
- Poached Salmon 35
- Apricot Salsa Salmon 37
- Orange Fish Fillets 39
- Fish with Tomatoes 41
- Shrimp Scampi 43
- Clam Chowder 45
- Lemon Pepper Tilapia with Asparagus 47
- Pesto Salmon with Vegetables 49
- Mustard Garlic Shrimps 51
- Mustard Crusted Salmon 53
- Five-Spice Tilapia 55
- Prosciutto-Wrapped Scallops 57
- Spicy Basil Shrimp 59
- Shrimps and Sausage Jambalaya Stew 60

Scallops with Sour Cream and Dill	62
Salmon with Lime Butter	63
Spicy Curried Shrimps	64
Smoked Trout	65
Salmon with Green Peppercorn Sauce	66
Coconut Curry Cod	68
Almond Crusted Tilapia	69
Buttered Bacon and Scallops	71
Lemony Shrimps in Hoisin Sauce	73
Garlic Butter Tilapia	75
Buttery Salmon with Onions and Carrots	77
Scalloped Potatoes with Salmon	79
Lemon-Herb Salmon	81
Orange Vinegar Salmon	83
Cod Stew	85
Fish and Beans	87
Asian Vegetables with a Salmon Blanket	89
Seafood Chowder	91
Shrimp Fra Diavolo	93
White Beans with Tuna	95
Coconut Clams	97
Seafood Gumbo	98
Jalapeño Spicy Tuna	100
Seasoned Large Shrimp	102
Mushrooms Snapper	104
Orange Cod	106
Cod with Shrimp Sauce	107

Beef Stroganoff

Preparation time: 15 minutes

Cooking time: 6 hours

Servings: 4 people

Ingredients:

- 4 minced garlic cloves
- 1 cup white mushrooms (approx. 10)
- 1 large chopped onion
- 3 tbsp. chopped parsley
- 2 cup bone broth
- 2 lbs. beef roast into small strips
- Pepper & salt to taste
- For Serving:
- 1 cucumber – peeled into long wide strips
- ½ cup coconut milk/cream
- 3 tbsp. Dijon mustard
- Garnish with parsley

- Salt to taste

Directions:

1. Arrange the strips of roast in the slow cooker. Stir in the salt, pepper, beef broth, mushrooms, garlic, and onion. Cook for 6 to 8 hours using the low-temperature setting.
2. When done, stir in the coconut cream, mustard, and salt. Cover a serving bowl with the cucumber noodles. Top it off with the stroganoff. Garnish with the parsley if desired.

Nutrition:

Calories: 462

Carbs: 4.0g

Fat: 36g

Protein: 26.0g

Cabbage & Corned Beef

Preparation time: 15 minutes

Cooking time: 8 hours

Servings: 4 people

Ingredients:

- 6 lb. corned beef
- 1 large head of cabbage
- 4 cups of water
- 1 celery bunch
- 1 small onion
- 4 carrots
- ½ tsp ground mustard
- ½ tsp ground coriander
- ½ tsp ground marjoram
- ½ tsp black pepper
- ½ tsp salt
- ½ tsp ground thyme

- ½ tsp allspice

Directions:

1. Dice the carrots, onions, and celery and toss them into the cooker. Pour in the water. Combine the spices, rub the beef, and arrange in the cooker. Cook on low within 7 hours.
2. Remove the top layer of cabbage. Wash and cut it into quarters until ready to cook. When the beef is done, add the cabbage, and cook for 1 hour on the low setting. Serve and enjoy.

Nutrition:

Calories: 583

Carbs: 13g

Fat: 40g

Protein: 42g

Chipotle Barbacoa – Mexican Barbecue

Preparation time: 15 minutes

Cooking time: 4-10 hours

Servings: 4 people

Ingredients:

- ½ cup beef/chicken broth
- 2 med. chilis in adobo (with the sauce, it's about 4 teaspoons)
- 3 lb. chuck roast/beef brisket
- 5 minced garlic cloves
- 2 tbsp lime juice
- 2 tbsp apple cider vinegar
- 2 tsp sea salt
- 2 tsp cumin
- 1 tbsp. dried oregano
- 1 tsp black pepper

- 2 whole bay leaves
- optional: ½ tsp ground cloves

Directions:

1. Mix the chilis in the sauce, and add the broth, garlic, ground cloves, pepper, cumin, salt, vinegar, and lime juice in a blender, mixing until smooth.
2. Chop the beef into two-inch chunks, and toss it in the slow cooker. Empty the puree on top. Toss in the two bay leaves.
3. Cook 4 to 6 hours on the high setting or 8 to 10 on low. Dispose of the bay leaves when the meat is done. Shred and stir into the juices to simmer for 5 to 10 minutes.

Nutrition: Calories: 242 Carbs: 2g Fat: 11g Protein: 32 g

Corned Beef Cabbage Rolls

Preparation time: 15 minutes

Cooking time: 6 hours

Servings: 4 people

Ingredients:

- 3 ½ lb. corned beef
- 15 large savoy cabbage leaves
- ¼ cup white wine
- ¼ cup coffee
- 1 large lemon
- 1 medium sliced onion
- 1 tbsp rendered bacon fat
- 1 tbsp sweetener
- 1 tbsp yellow mustard

- 2 tsp kosher salt
- 2 tsp Worcestershire sauce
- ¼ tsp cloves
- ¼ tsp allspice
- 1 large bay leaf
- 1 tsp mustard seeds
- 1 tsp whole peppercorns
- ½ tsp red pepper flakes

Directions:

1. Add the liquids, spices, and corned beef into the cooker. Cook 6 hours on the low setting. Prepare a pot of boiling water.

2. When the time is up, add the leaves and the sliced onion to the water for 2 to 3 minutes. Transfer the

leaves to a cold-water bath - blanching them for 3 to 4 minutes. Continue boiling the onion.

3. Use a paper towel to dry the leaves. Add the onions and beef, then roll up the cabbage leaves. Drizzle with freshly squeezed lemon juice.

Nutrition:

Calories: 481.4

Carbs: 4.2g

Protein: 34.87g

Fat: 25.38g

Cube Steak

Preparation time: 15 minutes

Cooking time: 8 hours

Servings: 4 people

Ingredients:

- 8 cubed steaks
- 1 ¾ tsp adobo seasoning/garlic salt
- 1 can tomato sauce
- 1 cup of water
- black pepper to taste
- ½ medium onion
- 1 small red pepper
- 1/3 cup green pitted olives (+) 2 tbsp. brine

Directions:

1. Slice the peppers and onions into ¼-inch strips. Sprinkle the steaks with the pepper and garlic salt as needed and place them in the slow cooker.

2. Fold in the peppers and onion and the water, sauce, and olives with the liquid/brine from the jar. Close the lid. Prepare using the low setting for 8 hours.

Nutrition:

Calories: 154

Carbs: 4g

Protein: 23.5g

Fat: 5.5g

Italian Meatballs & Zoodles

Preparation time: 15 minutes

Cooking time: 6 hours

Servings: 4 people

Ingredients:

- 1 medium spiraled zucchini
- 32 oz. beef stock
- 1 small diced onion
- 2 chopped celery ribs
- 1 chopped carrot
- 1 medium diced tomato
- 6 minced garlic cloves
- 1 ½ lb. ground beef
- 1 ½ tsp garlic salt

- ½ cup shredded parmesan cheese

- 1 large egg

- ½ tsp black pepper

- 4 tbsp. freshly chopped parsley

- 1 ½ tsp Onion powder

- 1 ½ tsp Sea salt

- 1 tsp Italian seasoning

- 1 tsp dried oregano

Directions:

1. Warm up the slow cooker with the low setting. Add the zucchini, beef stock, onion, celery, tomato, garlic salt, and carrot to the cooker. Cover with the lid.

2. Combine the beef, egg, parmesan, parsley, Italian seasonings, pepper, sea salt, oregano, garlic, and

onion powder in a mixing container. Mix and shape into 30 meatballs.

3. Warm up the oil using med-high heat in a frying pan. When it's hot, add the meatballs. Brown and toss into the cooker. Cook with the lid on within 6 hours on low. Serve.

Nutrition:

Calories: 129

Carbs: 3g

Fat.: 6g

Protein.: 15g

London Broil

Preparation time: 15 minutes

Cooking time: 4-6 hours

Servings: 4 people

Ingredients:

- 2 lb. London broil
- 1 tbsp. Dijon mustard
- 2 tbsp reduced sugar ketchup
- 2 tbsp coconut aminos or soy sauce
- ½ cup coffee
- ½ cup chicken broth
- ¼ cup white wine
- 2 tsp onion powder
- 2 tsp minced garlic

Directions:

1. Arrange the beef in the slow cooker. Cover both sides with the mustard, soy sauce, ketchup, and minced garlic.

2. Pour the liquids into the cooker and give it a sprinkle of the onion powder. Cook it for 4 to 6 hours. When it's ready, shred the meat. Combine with the juices. Serve and enjoy.

Nutrition:

Calories: 409

Carbs: 2.6g

Fat: 18.3g

Protein: 47.3g

Machaca - Mexican Pot Roast

Preparation time: 15 minutes

Cooking time: 7 hours

Servings: 4 people

Ingredients:

- 3 ½ lb. beef chuck roast
- 2 tsp granulated garlic
- ½ tsp ground coriander
- 1 tsp ground cumin
- 3 tbsp. bacon grease
- 1 tsp freshly ground black pepper
- Kosher salt
- 2 tbsp organic tomato paste

- 2 tbsp Worcestershire sauce

- 1 cup low-sodium beef/bone broth

- 2 cup fresh salsa

Directions:

1. Combine the garlic, cumin, salt, pepper, coriander, and cumin. Rub the beef all over. Melt the bacon grease in a heavy skillet using the med-high setting.

2. Brown the meat 2 minutes on each side. Arrange in the slow cooker and add the salsa, Worcestershire, tomato paste, and broth over the roast. Add the juices from the bacon and cover the slow cooker.

3. Cook 1 hour on the high setting. Lower the heat and cook until tender on the low power setting – about 6 to 8 hours.

4. When ready, shred, and remove any fat. Place the meat back into the juices of the slow cooker. Stir to coat and serve.

Nutrition:

Calories: 365

Carbs: 3g

Fat: 26g

Protein: 27g

Cranberry Pork Roast

Preparation time: 15 minutes

Cooking time: 6 hours

Servings: 4 people

Ingredients:

- 2 lb. pork shoulder, on the bone
- 1/4 cup dried minced onion
- 8 oz cranberry sauce, low-carb and sugar-free
- 1/4 cup raw honey

Directions:

1. Grease a 4-quart slow-cooker with a non-stick cooking spray and place the pork shoulder inside. Sprinkle with minced onion, then drizzle with honey, and top with the cranberry sauce.

2. Cover and seal the slow-cooker with its lid, then set the cooking timer for 5 to 6 hours. Allow to cook at a high heat setting, or until pork is cooked through and tender. Carve the meat and serve with the cooking juices alongside.

Nutrition:

Calories: 391.3

Carbs: 19.2g

Fats: 25g

Protein: 37g

Pulled Pork

Preparation time: 15 minutes

Cooking time: 6 hours

Servings: 2 people

Slow cooker size: 4-quart

Ingredients:

- 1 small pork roast, quartered
- 1 white onion, peeled and chopped
- 1 green pepper, sliced and chopped
- 3 tablespoons dry Italian seasoning

Directions:

1. Grease a 4-quart slow-cooker with a non-stick cooking spray and place the pork roast inside

it. Sprinkle with the Italian seasoning, then top with the onion and pepper.

2. Cover and seal the slow-cooker with its lid, then set the cooking timer for 5 to 6 hours. Allow to cook at a high heat setting, or until pork is cooked through and tender.

3. Shred the meat with forks and then serve between two roasted mushrooms caps with cream cheese.

Nutrition:

Calories: 214

Carbs: 4g

Fats: 12g

Protein: 21g

Balsamic Pork Tenderloin

Preparation time: 15 minutes

Cooking time: 6 hours

Servings: 4 people

Slow cooker size: 4-quart

Ingredients:

- 16 oz pork tenderloin
- 1/2 cup balsamic vinegar
- 2 tablespoon coconut aminos
- 1 tablespoon Worcestershire sauce
- 2 teaspoons minced garlic

Directions:

1. Grease a 4-quart slow-cooker with a non-stick cooking spray, place the pork inside, and sprinkle with the garlic.

2. Mix the remaining ingredients in a bowl, along with ½ teaspoon red pepper flakes. Pour this mixture over the pork, and seal the slow-cooker with its lid.

3. Set the cooking timer for 4 to 6 hours and cook at a low heat setting. Transfer the pork to a serving platter, drizzle with 1/2 cup of cooking liquid and carve to serve.

Nutrition:

Calories: 188

Carbs: 1.3g

Fats: 5.8g

Protein: 30.3g

Honey Mustard Barbecue Pork Ribs

Preparation time: 15 minutes

Cooking time: 5 hours

Servings: 4 people

Ingredients:

- 1 ½ lb. pork ribs, boneless
- 2 teaspoons garlic-and-herb seasoning blend
- 2 oz Dijon mustard
- 2 oz soy sauce
- 4 oz raw honey

Directions:

1. Put a large skillet pan on medium heat, and grease with a dash of olive oil. Cook the ribs in batches until they are nicely browned on all sides.

2. Drain the grease and transfer the browned pork ribs to a 4-quart slow cooker. Mix the remaining ingredients in a bowl.

3. Pour this mixture over pork ribs, then cover and seal the slow cooker with its lid. Set the cooking timer for 4 to 5 hours and cook at a high heat setting.

4. Transfer the pork ribs to a serving platter, skim any fat from the sauce, and drizzle the sauce over the chops. Serve hot.

Nutrition: Calories: 342 Carbs: 18.4g Fats: 20.2g Protein: 22.3g

Pork Chops with Broccoli

Preparation time: 15 minutes

Cooking time: 7 hours & 30 minutes

Servings: 4 people

Ingredients:

- 6 oz pork chops

- 1 medium-sized red onion, peeled and chopped

- 2 cups broccoli florets

- 4 tablespoons soy sauce

- 1 tablespoon sesame seeds

Directions:

1. Grease a 4-quarts slow-cooker with a non-stick cooking spray and place the pork, onion, soy sauce, and 1/2 cup water inside.

2. Cover and seal the slow cooker with its lid, and set the cooking timer for 7 hours, allowing it to cook at a high heat setting.

3. Add the broccoli and continue cooking for 20 to 30 minutes or until the broccoli is tender. Serve the meat, garnished with sesame seeds, with the vegetables and the sauce alongside.

Nutrition:

Calories: 293.9

Carbs: 5.7g

Carbs: 4.9g

Fats: 15g

Protein: 33.4g

Poached Salmon

Preparation time: 15 minutes

Cooking time: 2 hours

Servings: 4 people

Ingredients:

- 4 salmon fillets
- 1 medium-sized white onion, peeled and sliced
- 1 lemon, sliced
- 1/2 cup chicken broth
- 1 cup of water

Directions:

1. Place the ingredients in a 4-quart slow-cooker, holding back 4 lemon slices to garnish. Cover and

seal the slow cooker with its lid, then set the cooking timer for 2 hours on high. Serve hot, with the sauce alongside.

Nutrition:

Calories: 133

Carbs: 1.7g

Carbs: 0.96g

Fats: 3.9g

Protein: 22.9g

Apricot Salsa Salmon

Preparation time: 15 minutes

Cooking time: 1 hour & 30 minutes

Servings: 2 people

Ingredients:

- 8 oz wild salmon fillet
- 3 tablespoon apricot spread, sugar-free
- 1/4 cup Salsa Verde

Directions:

1. Grease a 4-quart slow-cooker with a non-stick cooking spray and place the salmon fillet into it. Stir the remaining ingredients together, and spread this mixture over the salmon.

2. Cover and seal the slow-cooker with its lid, and set the cooking timer for 1 to 1 1/2 hours. Allow to cook at a low heat setting or until salmon is cooked through. When done, flake the salmon fillet with forks and serve.

Nutrition:

Calories: 173.1

Carbs: 4.6g

Carbs: 4.2g

Fats: 6.3g

Protein: 27.1g

Orange Fish Fillets

Preparation time: 15 minutes

Cooking time: 2 hours

Servings: 4 people

Ingredients:

- 4 salmon fillets

- 4 oranges, segmented

- 1 tablespoon Dijon Mustard

- 1 tablespoon orange juice and a large piece of orange rind, sugar-free

- 1/2 cup apple cider vinegar

Directions:

1. Mix the vinegar, mustard, orange juice, orange rind, salt, and ground black pepper. Cut out 4 aluminum foil pieces, big enough to wrap around each fish fillet, then place a salmon fillet on each aluminum foil piece.

2. Spread prepared vinegar mixture over the top and top with the orange segments. Gently fold aluminum foil over each fillet and form a parcel by crimping the edges.

3. Place these parcels into a 4-quart slow cooker, then cover and seal the slow cooker with its lid. Set the cooking timer for 2 hours, allowing it to cook at a high heat setting.

4. Remove the aluminum packets with a tong, uncover fillets, flake with forks, and serve.

Nutrition: Calories: 120 Carbs: 2.7g Fats: 6.8g Protein: 19.1g

Fish with Tomatoes

Preparation time: 15 minutes

Cooking time: 1 hour & 30 minutes

Servings: 2 people

Ingredients:

- 6 oz cod
- 1 white onion, peeled and sliced
- 1 1/2 teaspoon minced garlic
- 1 can diced tomatoes
- 1/4 cup chicken broth

Directions:

1. Season the cod with a pinch of salt and pepper and red chili flakes. Mix the remaining ingredients, and place them into a 4-quart slow-cooker.

2. Gently place the seasoned cod on top, then cover and seal the slow-cooker with its lid, setting the cooking timer for 1 to 1 1/2 hours.
3. Allow to cook at a high heat setting or until fish is cooked through. Serve warm.

Nutrition:

Calories: 220

Carbs: 3.64g

Fats: 6.7g

Protein: 34.8g

Shrimp Scampi

Preparation time: 15 minutes

Cooking time: 2 hours & 30 minutes

Servings: 4 people

Ingredients:

- 16 oz shrimps, peeled, deveined, and rinsed
- 1 tablespoon minced garlic
- 2 tablespoon melted unsalted butter or olive oil
- 1 tablespoon lemon juice
- 3/4 cup chicken broth

Directions:

1. Mix all of the ingredients, apart from the shrimps. Season with salt and black pepper, and place in a 4-quarts slow-cooker. Add shrimps, mixing the ingredients gently together.

2. Cover and seal the slow cooker with its lid, and set the cooking timer for 2 1/2 hours. Allow to cook at a low heat setting or until shrimps are cooked through. Garnish with cheese and serve immediately.

Nutrition:

Calories: 256

Carbs: 2.1g

Fats: 14.7g

Protein: 23.3g

Clam Chowder

Preparation time: 15 minutes

Cooking time: 4-6 hours

Servings: 4 people

Ingredients:

- 1 ¼ lb. baby clams, with juice
- 1 cup of chopped onion
- 1 cup chopped celery
- 1 teaspoon dried thyme
- 2 cups coconut cream, full-fat
- 2 cups chicken broth

Directions:

1. Grease a 4-quarts slow-cooker with a non-stick cooking spray and place all ingredients inside. Flavor it with a pinch of salt and ground black pepper.

2. Cover and seal the slow-cooker with its lid, and set the cooking timer for 4 to 6 hours. Allow cooking at a low heat setting or until cooked. Serve immediately.

Nutrition:

Calories: 391

Carbs: 5g

Fats: 29g

Protein: 27g

Lemon Pepper Tilapia with Asparagus

Preparation time: 15 minutes

Cooking time: 3 hours

Servings: 4 people

Ingredients:

- 6 Tilapia fillets
- 1 bundle of asparagus
- 4 teaspoons lemon-pepper seasoning
- 3 tablespoons unsalted butter
- 1/2 cup lemon juice

Directions:

1. Cut out 6 aluminum foil pieces, each big enough to wrap a tilapia fillet. Put each fillet on a piece of aluminum foil, then evenly sprinkle with lemon-pepper seasoning and lemon juice.

2. Top each fillet with a knob of butter, then place the asparagus spears on top. Gently fold the aluminum foil over each fillet, and form a parcel by crimping the edges.
3. Place these parcels into a 4-quart slow cooker, then cover and seal the slow cooker with its lid. Set the cooking timer for 3 hours, cook at a high heat setting or until fillets are cooked through.
4. Remove the parcels with a tong, unwrap the fillets, flake the fish with forks, and serve.

Nutrition:

Calories: 320

Carbs: 10g

Fats: 24g

Protein: 60g

Pesto Salmon with Vegetables

Preparation time: 15 minutes

Cooking time: 2-3 hours

Servings: 2 people

Ingredients:

- 2 salmon fillets
- 8 oz fresh green beans, trimmed
- 4 teaspoons basil pesto
- 10 cherry tomatoes, quartered
- 3 lemons, juiced

Directions:

1. Grease a 4-quart slow cooker with a non-stick cooking spray and place the cherry tomatoes and green beans inside.
2. Rub the salmon fillets with salt and black pepper, and place on top of the vegetables. Mix the pesto and the

lemon juice, then drizzle over the salmon fillets and vegetables.

3. Cover and seal the slow cooker with its lid, and set the cooking timer for 2 to 3 hours. Allow to cook at a low heat setting or until fillets are cooked through. Serve fish fillet and vegetables with cooked cauliflower rice.

Nutrition:

Calories: 435

Carbs: 5g

Fats: 26g

Protein: 33g

Mustard Garlic Shrimps

Preparation time: 5 minutes

Cooking time: 2 hours and 30 minutes

Servings: 4 people

Ingredients:

- 1 teaspoon olive oil
- 3 tablespoons garlic, minced
- 1-pound shrimp, shelled and deveined
- 1 teaspoon Dijon mustards
- Salt and pepper to taste
- Parsley for garnish

Directions:

1. Heat-up olive oil in a skillet and sauté the garlic until fragrant and slightly browned. Transfer to the slow

cooker and place the shrimps and Dijon mustard. Stir to combine.

2. Season with salt and pepper to taste. Close the lid and cook on low for 2 hours or high for 30 minutes. Once done, sprinkle with parsley.

Nutrition:

Calories: 138

Carbs: 3.2g

Protein: 23.8g

Fat: 2.7g

Mustard Crusted Salmon

Preparation time: 3 minutes

Cooking time: 4 hours

Servings: 4 people

Ingredients:

- 4 pieces of salmon fillets
- salt and pepper to taste
- 2 teaspoons lemon juice
- 2 tablespoons stone-ground mustard
- ¼ cup full sour cream

Directions:

1. Flavor the salmon fillets with salt and pepper to taste. Sprinkle with lemon juice. Rub the stone-ground mustard all over the fillets.

2. Place inside the slow cooker and cook on high for 2 hours or on low for 4 hours. An hour before the cooking time, pour in the sour cream on top of the fish. Continue cooking until the fish becomes flaky.

Nutrition:

Calories: 74

Carbs: 4.2g

Protein: 25.9g

Fat:13.8g

Five-Spice Tilapia

Preparation time: 3 minutes

Cooking time: 5 hours

Servings: 4 people

Ingredients:

- 4 tilapia fillets
- 1 teaspoon Chinese five-spice powder
- 1 tablespoon sesame oil
- ¼ cup gluten-free soy sauce
- 3 scallions, thinly sliced

Directions:

1. Season the tilapia fillets with the Chinese five-spice powder. Place sesame oil in the slow cooker and arrange the fish on top. Cook on high within 2 hours and low for 4 hours.

2. Halfway through the cooking time, flip the fish to slightly brown on the other side. Once cooking time is done, add the soy sauce and scallion and continue cooking for another hour.

Nutrition:

Calories: 153

Carbs: 0.9g

Protein: 25.8g

Fat: 5.6g

Prosciutto-Wrapped Scallops

Preparation time: 3 minutes

Cooking time: 3 hours

Servings: 4 people

Ingredients:

- 12 large scallops, rinsed and patted dry
- Salt and pepper to taste
- 1 ¼ oz. prosciutto, cut into 12 long strips
- 1 tablespoon extra-virgin olive oil
- 1 tablespoon lemon juice

Directions:

1. Sprinkle individual scallops with salt and pepper to taste. Wrap prosciutto around the scallops. Set aside.

2. Add oil to the slow cooker and arrange on top the bacon-wrapped scallops. Pour over the lemon juice. Cook on low within 1 hour or on high for 3 hours.
3. Halfway through the cooking time, flip the scallops. Continue cooking until scallops are done.

Nutrition:

Calories: 113

Carbs: 5g

Protein: 15.9g

Fat:8 g

Spicy Basil Shrimp

Preparation time: 3 minutes

Cooking time: 2 hours

Servings: 4 people

Ingredients:

- 1-pound raw shrimp, shelled and deveined
- Salt and pepper to taste
- 1 tablespoon butter
- ¼ cup packed fresh basil leaves
- ¼ teaspoon cayenne pepper

Directions:

1. Add all ingredients to the slow cooker. Give a stir. Cook on high within 30 minutes or on low for 2 hours.

Nutrition: Calories: 144 Carbs: 1.4g Protein: 23.4g Fat: 6.2g

Shrimps and Sausage Jambalaya Stew

Preparation time: 5 minutes

Cooking time: 3 hours

Servings: 4 people

Ingredients:

- 1 teaspoon canola oil
- 8 oz. andouille sausage, cut into slices
- 1 bag frozen bell pepper plus onion mix
- 1 can chicken broth
- 8 oz. shrimps, shelled and deveined

Directions:

1. In a skillet, heat the oil and sauté the sausages until the sausages have rendered their fat. Set aside. Pour the vegetable mix into the slow cooker.

Scallops with Sour Cream and Dill

Preparation time: 3 minutes

Cooking time: 2 hours

Servings: 4 people

Ingredients:

- 1 ¼ pounds scallops
- Salt and pepper to taste
- 3 teaspoons butter
- ¼ cup sour cream
- 1 tablespoon fresh dill

Directions:

1. Add all ingredients into the slow cooker. Give a good stir to combine everything. Cook on high within 30 minutes or on low for 2 hours.

Nutrition: Calories: 152 Carbs: 4.3g Protein: 18.2g Fat: 5.7g

2. Add in the sausages and pour the chicken broth in the shrimps last. Cook on low within 1 hour o low for 3 hours.

Nutrition:

Calories: 316

Carbs: 6.3

Protein: 32.1g

Fat: 25.6g

Salmon with Lime Butter

Preparation time: 3 minutes

Cooking time: 4 hours

Servings: 4 people

Ingredients:

- 1-pound salmon fillet cut into 4 portions
- 1 tablespoon butter, melted
- Salt and pepper to taste
- 2 tablespoons lime juice
- ½ teaspoon lime zest, grated

Directions:

1. Add all ingredients to the slow cooker. Close the lid. Cook on high within 2 hours and low for 4 hours.

Nutrition: Calories: 206 Carbs: 1.8g Protein:23.7 g Fat: 15.2g

Spicy Curried Shrimps

Preparation time: 3 minutes

Cooking time: 2 hours

Servings: 4 people

Ingredients:

- 1 ½ pounds shrimp, shelled and deveined
- 1 tablespoon ghee or butter, melted
- 1 tablespoon curry powder
- 1 teaspoon cayenne pepper
- Salt and pepper to taste

Directions:

1. Place all ingredients in the slow cooker. Give a stir to incorporate everything. Cook on low within 2 hours or on high for 30 minutes.

Nutrition: Calories: 207 Carbs:2.2 g Protein: 35.2g Fat: 10.5g

Smoked Trout

Preparation time: 3 minutes

Cooking time: 2 hours

Servings: 4

Ingredients:

- 2 tablespoons of liquid smoke
- 2 tablespoons olive oil
- 4 oz. smoked trout; skin removed then flaked
- Salt and pepper to taste
- 2 tablespoons mustard

Directions:

1. Place all ingredients in the slow cooker. Cook on high within 1 hour or low for 2 hours until the trout flakes have absorbed the sauce.

Nutrition: Calories: 116 Carbs: 1.5g Protein: 7.2g Fat: 9.2g

Salmon with Green Peppercorn Sauce

Preparation time: 5 minutes

Cooking time: 3 hours

Servings: 4 people

Ingredients:

- 1 ¼ pounds salmon fillets, skin removed and cut into 4 portions
- Salt and pepper to taste
- 4 teaspoons unsalted butter
- ¼ cup lemon juice
- 1 teaspoon green peppercorns in vinegar

Directions:

1. Flavor the salmon fillets with salt plus pepper to taste. In a skillet, heat the butter and sear the salmon fillets for 2 minutes on each side.

2. Transfer in the slow cooker and pour the lemon juice and green peppercorns. Adjust the seasoning by adding in more salt or pepper depending on your taste. Cook on high within 1 hour or low for 3 hours.

Nutrition:

Calories: 255

Carbs: 2.3g

Protein: 37.4g

Fat: 13.5g

Coconut Curry Cod

Preparation time: 3 minutes

Cooking time: 4 hours

Servings: 4 people

Ingredients:

- 4 pieces of cod fillets
- Salt and pepper to taste
- 1 ½ cups coconut milk
- 2 teaspoons curry paste
- 2 teaspoons grated ginger

Directions:

1. Place all ingredients in the slow cooker. Give a good stir. Cook on high within 2 hours or on low for 4 hours. Garnish with chopped cilantro if desired.

Nutrition: Calories: 296 Carbs: 6.7g Protein: 20.1g Fat: 22.8g

Almond Crusted Tilapia

Preparation time: 5 minutes

Cooking time: 4 hours

Servings: 4 people

Ingredients:

- 2 tablespoons olive oil
- 1 cup chopped almonds
- ¼ cup ground flaxseed
- 4 tilapia fillets
- Salt and pepper to taste

Directions:

1. Arrange the bottom of the slow cooker with a foil. Grease the foil with olive oil. In a mixing bowl, combine the almonds and flaxseed.

2. Season the tilapia with salt and pepper to taste. Dredge the tilapia fillets with the almond and flaxseed mixture.
3. Place neatly in the foil-lined slow cooker—cook on high within 2 hours and low for 4 hours.

Nutrition:

Calories: 233

Carbs: 4.6g

Protein: 25.5g

Fat: 13.3g

Buttered Bacon and Scallops

Preparation time: 5 minutes

Cooking time: 2 hours

Servings: 4 people

Ingredients:

- 1 tablespoon butter
- 2 cloves of garlic, chopped
- 24 scallops, rinsed and patted dry
- Salt and pepper to taste
- 1 cup bacon, chopped

Directions:

1. In a skillet, heat the butter and sauté the garlic until fragrant and lightly browned. Transfer to a slow cooker and add the scallops.

2. Season with salt and pepper to taste. Cook on high within 45 minutes or low for 2 hours.

3. Meanwhile, cook the bacon until the fat has rendered and crispy. Sprinkle the cooked scallops with crispy bacon.

Nutrition:

Calories: 261

Carbs: 4.9 g

Protein: 24.7 g

Fat: 14.3 g

Lemony Shrimps in Hoisin Sauce

Preparation time: 3 minutes

Cooking time: 2 hours

Servings: 4 people

Ingredients:

- 1/3 cup hoisin sauce
- ½ cup lemon juice, freshly squeezed
- 1 ½ pounds shrimps, shelled and deveined
- Salt and pepper to taste
- 2 tablespoon cilantro leaves, chopped

Directions:

1. Into the slow cooker, place the hoisin sauce, lemon juice, and shrimps. Season with salt and pepper to taste.
2. Mix to incorporate all ingredients. Cook on high within 30 minutes or on low for 2 hours. Garnish with cilantro leaves.

Nutrition:

Calories: 228

Carbs: 6.3g

Protein: 35.8g

Fat: 3.2g

Garlic Butter Tilapia

Preparation time: 15 minutes

Cooking time: 2 hours

Servings: 4 people

Ingredients:

- 2 tablespoons butter, at room temperature
- 2 garlic cloves, minced
- 2 teaspoons flat parsley, chopped
- 4 tilapia fillets
- 1 lemon, cut into wedges
- Salt and pepper to taste
- Cooking spray

Directions:

1. Put a sheet of aluminum foil on a work surface. Place fillets in the middle. Place in a slow cooker. Season generously with salt and pepper.

2. Mix butter with minced garlic and chopped parsley. Evenly spread mixture over each fillet. Wrap foil around fish, sealing all sides—cook on high for 2 hours. Serve with lemon wedges.

Nutrition:

Calories: 89

Fat: 9.8 g

Carbs: 0.5 g

Protein: 8.4g

Buttery Salmon with Onions and Carrots

Preparation time: 15 minutes

Cooking time: 9 hours

Servings: 4 people

Ingredients:

- 4 salmon fillets
- 4 tablespoons butter
- 4 onions, chopped
- 16 oz. baby carrots
- 3 cloves garlic, minced
- Salt and pepper

Directions:

1. Dissolve the butter in the microwave, and pour into the slow cooker. Add onions, garlic, and baby carrots.

Cover and cook for 6-7 hours on low, occasionally stirring until vegetables begin to caramelize.

2. Place fillet over vegetables in the slow cooker, and season with salt and pepper. Cover and cook on low for 1-2 hours until salmon flakes. Serve on a serving plate, and top with onion mixture.

Nutrition:

Calories: 367

Fat: 22 g

Carbs: 12.2 g

Protein: 39g

Scalloped Potatoes with Salmon

Preparation time: 15 minutes

Cooking time: 7-8 hours

Servings: 4 people

Ingredients:

- 3 tablespoons all-purpose flour
- 1 10¾-ounce can of cream of mushroom soup
- 5 medium-sized potatoes, peeled and sliced
- 1 16-ounce can of salmon, drained and flaked
- ½ cup chopped onions
- ¼ cup of water
- Salt and pepper
- Cooking spray

Directions:

1. Generously spray the slow cooker bottom and sides with cooking spray. Place half of the potatoes in a

slow cooker. Sprinkle with half of the flour, then season with salt and pepper.

2. Cover with half the flaked salmon, then sprinkle with half the onions. Repeat layers. Combine soup and water.

3. Pour over top of potato and salmon mixture. Cover and cook on low within 7-8 hours or until potatoes are tender.

Nutrition:

Calories: 367

Fat: 22g

Carbs: 5.2g

Protein: 39g

Lemon-Herb Salmon

Preparation time: 15 minutes

Cooking time: 3 hours

Servings: 4 people

Ingredients:

- 2 pounds skin-on salmon
- 2 cups of water
- 1 tablespoon crushed garlic
- 1 tablespoon lemon
- 1 cup onion
- 1 teaspoon black pepper
- 2 tablespoons dried parsley
- 3 tablespoons butter
- ¼ cup dill
- 1 teaspoon salt
- Fresh parsley, dill, and lemon slices for garnishing

Directions:

1. Combine the water, garlic, lemon juice, onion, black pepper, parsley, butter, dill, and salt in the slow cooker and cook on high for 30 minutes.
2. Place the salmon in the slow cooker and cook for about 2 hours and 30 minutes. Garnish with some fresh parsley, dill, and lemon slices.

Nutrition:

Calories: 418

Fat: 25.4 g

Carbs: 2 g

Protein: 46g

Orange Vinegar Salmon

Preparation time: 15 minutes

Cooking time: 2 hours

Servings: 2 people

Ingredients:

- 1 tablespoon Dijon mustard
- 3 tablespoons orange juice
- ¼ cup apple cider vinegar
- 4 salmon fillets
- Salt and pepper to taste
- 4 oranges, peeled and segmented

Directions:

1. In a bowl, mix the mustard, orange juice, and apple cider vinegar. Layout 4 aluminum foil pieces big enough to wrap one fillet each.

2. Place each fillet on a piece of aluminum foil, and season with salt and pepper. Top with some sauce and orange segments.

3. Gently fold the aluminum foil over each fillet, and make a closed pack by crimping the edges. Place them in a slow cooker.

4. Cook on high for 2 hours. Being mindful of the steam, open the foil packets. Flake the fish with forks, and serve.

Nutrition:

Calories: 123

Fat: 6.8g

Carbs: 2.8g

Protein: 19g

Cod Stew

Preparation time: 15 minutes

Cooking time: 6-8 hours & 40 minutes

Servings: 2 people

Ingredients:

- 2 medium potatoes, finely chopped
- 1/3 cup corn kernels
- ¼ cup lima beans
- 1 small onion, chopped
- ½ stalk celery, sliced
- 1 small carrot, chopped
- 1 clove garlic, minced
- ½ bay leaf
- ¼ teaspoon crushed rosemary
- Salt and pepper to taste
- ¼ cup chicken broth
- 3 oz. condensed cream of celery soup

- ¼ cup white wine
- ½ pound cod fillets, cut in pieces, bones removed
- 4 oz. diced tomatoes, drained
- ½ cup evaporated milk

Directions:

1. Combine the potatoes, corn, lima beans, onion, celery, carrot, garlic, bay leaf, rosemary, salt and pepper, chicken broth, celery soup, and white wine slow cooker. Mix well.

2. Cover, and cook on low within 6–8 hours, until the potatoes are tender. Now, remove the bay leaf and add the cod, tomatoes, and milk. Mix well—cover and cook for 35 to 40 minutes. Serve.

Nutrition: Calories: 168 Fat: 2g Carbs: 29g Protein: 14g

Fish and Beans

Preparation time: 15 minutes

Cooking time: 7 hours & 5 minutes

Servings: 4 people

Ingredients:

- 4 tablespoons olive oil
- 1 clove garlic, crushed
- 1-pound small white beans, soaked overnight, drained
- 6 cups of water
- 2 cups tomatoes, chopped
- 2 to 3 cans white tuna in water, drained, flaked
- 1½ teaspoons dried basil
- salt
- ground black pepper

Directions:

1. Sauté the garlic in oil for a minute over medium heat to flavor the oil. Pour the oil into the slow cooker and top with the beans and water.
2. Cook everything on high for 1 hour, and then on low for 4 to 7 hours. Mix in the rest of the ingredients and cook for another 5 minutes. Transfer everything to a bowl and serve.

Nutrition:

Calories: 250

Fat: 3 g

Carbs: 15 g

Protein: 10g

Asian Vegetables with a Salmon Blanket

Preparation time: 15 minutes

Cooking time: 2-3 hours

Servings: 4 people

Ingredients:

- 10 oz. salmon fillets
- Salt and pepper, to taste
- 1 package frozen Asian stir fry vegetable blend
- 2 tablespoons soy sauce
- 2 tablespoons honey
- 2 tablespoons lemon juice
- 1 teaspoon sesame seeds (optional)

Directions:

1. Season the salmon with salt and pepper. Mix the soy sauce, honey, and lemon juice in a separate bowl. Put the Asian vegetables in the bottom of a slow cooker.

2. Lay the fillets over the vegetables and then pour the soy sauce mixture over everything; if you're using the sesame seeds, sprinkle them on top now.

3. Cook everything on low for 2 to 3 hours. Transfer the vegetables and fish to a plate and cover with the sauce from the slow cooker.

Nutrition:

Calories: 110

Fat: 3g

Carbs: 18g

Protein: 3g

Seafood Chowder

Preparation time: 15 minutes

Cooking time: 7 hours

Servings: 4 people

Ingredients:

- 2 pounds frozen fish filets, thawed
- ¼ pound bacon or streaky salt pork, diced
- 1 medium onion, chopped
- 4 medium red-skinned potatoes, peeled, cubed
- 2 cups of water
- 1 to 1½ teaspoons kosher salt
- ¼ teaspoon pepper
- 1 can (12 oz.) evaporated milk

Directions:

1. Cut the fillets into bite-sized chunks and place them in the slow cooker. Sauté the bacon or pork over medium heat until golden brown. Add the onions and sauté some more.
2. Drain the oil and add the sautéed mixture to the slow cooker. Add the rest of the ingredients, except the milk, and cook everything on low for 5 to 6 hours.
3. Pour the milk into the cooker and continue cooking for another hour. Transfer everything to a bowl and serve.

Nutrition:

Calories: 174

Fat: 7g

Carbs: 15g

Protein: 8g

Shrimp Fra Diavolo

Preparation time: 15 minutes

Cooking time: 3 hours & 25 minutes

Servings: 2 people

Ingredients:

- 1 tablespoon coconut oil
- 1 medium onion, diced
- 6 cloves garlic, minced
- 1 teaspoon red pepper flakes
- ¼ cup chicken or vegetable broth
- 3 large tomatoes, grilled, peeled, and diced
- 1 tablespoon minced parsley
- ½ teaspoon freshly ground black pepper
- ½ pound medium-size shrimp shelled
- Chopped Chives for serving

Directions:

1. Heat-up oil in a pan over medium heat. Add the onion, garlic, and pepper and sauté until the onions are translucent, for about 10 minutes.
2. Transfer to the slow cooker and add the broth, tomatoes, parsley, and black pepper. Cook for 2 to 3 hours on low.
3. Add the shrimp and cook for 15 minutes on high or until the shrimp has changed color and has become opaque. Put the chopped chives before serving, if desired.

Nutrition:

Calories: 278

Fat: 9.3g

Carbs: 20.3g

Protein: 26.3g

White Beans with Tuna

Preparation time: 15 minutes

Cooking time: 10 hours & 30 minutes

Servings: 4 people

Ingredients:

- 2 tablespoons garlic-infused oil
- 1-pound small white beans, soaked overnight and drained
- 6 cups of water
- 2 cups chopped tomatoes
- 2 6 ½ oz. can white tuna in water, drained and flaked
- 1 ½ teaspoon dried basil
- Salt and pepper, to taste

Directions:

1. Combine the garlic-infused oil with the beans and 6 cups water in the slow cooker. Cover and cook for 2

hours on high. Continue cooking 8 hours on low. Add remaining fixings and cook within 30 minutes on high. Serve.

Nutrition:

Calories: 238

Fat: 4.4 g

Carbs: 20 g

Protein: 27g

Coconut Clams

Preparation time: 15 minutes

Cooking time: 6 hours

Servings: 2 people

Ingredients:

- ¼ cup of coconut milk
- 2 eggs, whisked
- 1 tablespoon olive oil
- 10 oz. canned clams, chopped
- 1 green bell pepper, chopped
- 1 yellow onion, chopped
- Salt and black pepper to taste

Directions:

1. Combine all the fixings in the slow cooker. Cover, and cook on low for 6 hours. Divide among serving bowls or plates and enjoy!

Nutrition: Calories: 271 Fat: 4.2g Carbs: 16g Protein: 7.6g

Seafood Gumbo

Preparation time: 15 minutes

Cooking time: 5 hours

Servings: 4 people

Ingredients:

- 8-10 bacon strips, sliced
- 2 stalks celery, sliced
- 1 medium onion, sliced
- 1 green pepper, chopped
- 2 garlic cloves, minced
- 2 cups chicken broth
- 1 14-ounce can dice tomatoes, undrained
- 2 tablespoons Worcestershire sauce
- 2 teaspoons salt
- 1 teaspoon dried thyme leaves
- 1-pound large raw shrimp, peeled, deveined
- 1 pound fresh or frozen crabmeat

- 1 10-ounce box frozen okra, thawed and sliced into ½-inch pieces

Directions:

1. Cook the bacon in your skillet on medium heat. When crisp, drain and transfer to a slow cooker. Drain off drippings, leaving just enough to coat the skillet.
2. Sauté celery, onion, green pepper, and garlic until vegetables are tender, then transfer the sautéed vegetables to the slow cooker. Add the broth, tomatoes, Worcestershire sauce, salt, and thyme.
3. Cover and cook within 4 hours on low or for 2 hours on high. Add the shrimp, crabmeat, and okra. Cover and cook within 1 hour longer on low or 30 minutes longer on high.

Nutrition: Calories: 273 Fat: 8g Carbs: 11g Protein: 4g

Jalapeño Spicy Tuna

Preparation time: 15 minutes

Cooking time: 5 hours

Servings: 2 people

Ingredients:

- 1 tablespoon olive oil
- 2-3 jalapeño peppers, membrane and seeds removed and finely diced
- 1 red bell peppers, trimmed and chopped
- 1 garlic clove, minced
- ¾ pound tuna loin, cubed
- Salt and black pepper

Directions:

1. Grease the inside cooking surface of the slow cooker with olive oil. In it, combine all the ingredients except the tuna. Cook on low for 3 hours and 45 minutes.
2. Season the tuna with salt and pepper. Open the lid and add the tuna, spooning some of the sauce over the fish—cook on high for 15 minutes. Serve hot.

Nutrition:

Calories: 202

Fat: 4.1g

Carbs: 16.3g

Protein: 4.5g

Seasoned Large Shrimp

Preparation time: 15 minutes

Cooking time: 2 hours & 30 minutes

Servings: 4 people

Ingredients:

- ½ cup chicken broth
- ½ cup white wine (optional; if using white wine, reduce chicken broth to ¼ cup)
- 2 tablespoons olive oil
- 2 teaspoons garlic, chopped
- 2 teaspoons parsley, minced
- 1-pound large raw shrimp, thawed

Directions:

1. Place all the fixings except the shrimp in your slow cooker and mix. Place the shrimp into the mixture

and cook everything on low for 2 hours and 30 minutes.

2. Remove the shrimp and place in a bowl. Stir the mixture one last time and then pour over the shrimp. Serve and enjoy.

Nutrition:

Calories: 130

Fat: 1 g

Carbs: 15 g

Protein: 4g

Mushrooms Snapper

Preparation time: 15 minutes

Cooking time: 6 hours

Servings: 4 people

Ingredients:

- 1 cup sour cream
- 1 onion, diced
- ¼ cup almond milk
- 1 tsp salt
- 7 oz cremini mushrooms
- 1 tsp ground thyme
- 1 tbsp ground paprika
- 1 tsp ground coriander
- 1 tsp kosher salt
- 1 tbsp lemon juice
- 1 tsp butter
- 1 lb. snapper, chopped

- 1 tsp lemon zest

Directions:

1. Season the snapper with thyme, paprika, coriander, salt, lemon zest, and lemon juice in a bowl. Cover the snapper and marinate it for 10 minutes.
2. Grease the insert of the slow cooker with butter and add a snapper mixture. Add cremini mushrooms, onion, almond milk, and sour cream.
3. Put the cooker's lid on and set the cooking time to 6 hours on low. Serve warm.

Nutrition:

Calories: 248

Fat: 6.3g

Carbs: 31.19g

Protein: 20g

Orange Cod

Preparation time: 15 minutes

Cooking time: 3 hours

Servings: 4 people

Ingredients:

- 1-pound cod fillet, chopped
- 2 oranges, chopped
- 1 tablespoon maple syrup
- 1 cup of water
- 1 garlic clove, diced
- 1 teaspoon ground black pepper

Directions:

1. Mix cod with ground black pepper and transfer to the slow cooker. Add garlic, water, maple syrup, and oranges. Close the lid and cook the meal on high for 3 hours.

Nutrition: Calories: 150 Protein: 21.2g Carbs: 14.8g Fat: 1.2g

Cod with Shrimp Sauce

Preparation time: 15 minutes

Cooking time: 2 hours

Servings: 4 people

Ingredients:

- 1 lb. cod fillets, cut into medium pieces
- 2 tbsp parsley, chopped
- 4 oz. breadcrumbs
- 2 tsp lemon juice
- 2 eggs, whisked
- 2 oz. butter, melted
- ½ pint milk
- ½ pint shrimp sauce
- Salt and black pepper to the taste

Directions:

1. Toss fish with crumbs, parsley, salt, black pepper, and lemon juice in a suitable bowl. Add butter, milk, egg, and fish mixture to the insert of the slow cooker.

2. Put the cooker's lid on and set the cooking time to 2 hours on high. Serve warm.

Nutrition:

Calories: 231

Fat: 3g

Carbs: 10g

Protein: 5g

www.ingramcontent.com/pod-product-compliance
Lightning Source LLC
Chambersburg PA
CBHW071112030426
42336CB00013BA/2051